GLUTEN FREE TAX RELIEF

WHY IS GLUTEN-FREE SO EXPENSIVE AND HOW TO GET MONEY BACK

Written by:
Kenneth & Katherine Henry

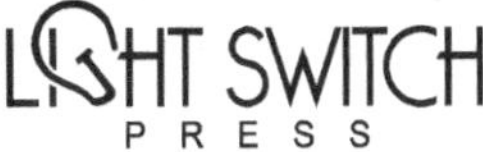

Published by:

Light Switch Press
PO Box 272847
Fort Collins, CO 80527

www.lightswitchpress.com

Gluten Free Tax Relief

ISBN: 978-1-944255-39-8

Copyright © 2017 by Kenneth & Katherine Henry

Cover Concept: Nalen Henry-Newton

Cover Design: Light Switch Press

Printed in the United States of America

DEDICATION

John David, the oldest son, we are proud of your time in the military and your service to this great country. We are so proud of the man you have become and will continue to be; you bring a smile to our faces always.

Michael, the middle son, we are proud of everything you have accomplished in life. You take the hard times and make them better, you hold your head up when things aren't always at their brightest and your smile lights up a room for all to see. You have the biggest heart we've ever seen.

Nalen, the youngest son, you are an intelligent young man with a future of being and doing whatever it is you set your mind to. Shoot for the stars and you will achieve the greatness you seek. Your smile is infectious as is your personality; may you never lose your glow.

By the way, we are still waiting for grandchildren!!

Ken & Katherine

TABLE OF CONTENTS

FOREWORD

I have known Ken and Katherine for quite a while and didn't quite understand the whole Gluten-Free money issue until my wife went through something similar. We now have to be Gluten-Free in our household and the cost is pretty high, especially with a child at home since kids can be pretty picky eaters.

When Ken and Katherine first showed me their idea for a book, I have to be honest, I thought it was cool, but not really sure about it, until I looked into what they was talking about and it made a lot of sense.

Ken and Katherine have put together a book that makes sense and provides a ledger to help keep track of everything you spend and the price difference, so at the end of the year all the numbers are there. This is something that will be used in my household and I hope many others.

Michael Neufeld

Chief Nurse West Point Emergency Room

PREFACE

This book is all about helping people with celiac disease or gluten allergies to save money. Gluten-free items cost $$$$, the first question we asked ourselves was, "WHY?" Upon further research, we found that we could get some of the money back that we had spent when we file taxes. We may have to spend the money up front, but why not collect monies back at the end of the year? Why should we suffer for having issues we can't control?

This book will help to guide you in the right direction. We show you how to get money back as well as provide a ledger to help you keep track weekly. This way when filing taxes at the end of the year, you have all the information at your fingertips – readily accessible and accurate.

INTRODUCTION

My wife Katherine discovered she had celiac disease a couple of years ago. She was having all kinds of medical issues with no answers and then she had an endoscopy. It came back pretty nasty looking – everything inside was rotted and pretty gross looking. That day, we cleaned out everything in the house and went shopping for gluten-free foods only to discover the cost was outrageous.

Due to Katherine's issue and changing our diet, we discovered the costs of gluten-free and a way around it. We are here to share that knowledge and help save people money (or at least get some of it back).

CHAPTER ONE
Gluten Free Tax Relief

Questions ? ? ? ? ?

Why are gluten free (GF) foods so much more expensive?

Why are GF foods so hard to locate?

Is there any way to save money and eat GF?

I will answer these questions and more. Please enjoy the read and learning how you too can save money.

Hello, my name is Ken and my wife Katherine was having all kinds of medical issues that no one could give an answer to until the day she was given an endoscopy and we discovered she had celiac! The very first question we asked was, "What is celiac?" This was a new word for both of us and of course I joked, "Yep you're a silly act alright – ha ha ha!" Needless to say, she didn't laugh as she had already looked it up and was very upset. So I had to do some reading myself…and do some apologizing to say the least.

Celiac disease is a serious genetic autoimmune disorder where the ingestion of gluten leads to damage in the small intestine. It is estimated to affect 1 in 100 people worldwide. Over two million Americans are undiagnosed and are at risk for long-term health complications. When people with celiac disease eat gluten (a protein found in wheat, rye and barley), their body mounts an immune response that attacks the small intestine. These attacks lead to damage on the villi, small fingerlike projections that line the small intestine, that promote nutrient absorption. When the villi get damaged, nutrients **cannot be absorbed** properly into the body. The only treatment currently for celiac disease is a strict, gluten-free diet. Most patients report symptom improvement within a few weeks, although intestinal healing may take several years. Celiac disease is hereditary, meaning that it runs in families. People with a first-degree relative with celiac disease (parent, child, and sibling) have a 1 in 10 chance of developing celiac disease.

So, Katherine's results were nasty. There was black rot in her lining that showed in the pictures we received from the doctor. It was NOT a pretty sight. The joke was over – my wife had a serious medical condition and we were bound and determined to find answers like what was causing the issues and how to combat it like warriors on a battlefield; and we would be triumphant in our journey…

The first step was to figure out the whole shopping for celiac thing, which wasn't an easy thing to do since no one around us had a clue what we were even asking. They looked at us like we had foreign objects growing out of our foreheads. The words "gluten free" meant almost nothing to anyone – like we were making up our own language.

So we eventually started finding gluten free foods, but there was another issue, the taste (YUCK!). It was like eating cardboard without the flavor and the texture was horrible. But we pushed through for a couple of reasons: first, we knew we had to; secondly, my lovely wife emptied out and gave away ALL the food in the house as soon as she found out about the wheat, barley, etc..; and third, of course is that I didn't want to go hungry.

The next issue besides the taste of the food available was the cost. We are a military family and don't make that much money. Our first trip to the store cost us over $700, I almost flipped. We walked out with only 4 bags of groceries for $700…who sets these prices?

So we suffered and I do mean suffered. We were always broke and eating crap they called food. Although the taste has gotten much better, the prices, well that's another story altogether.

With my wife, being tenacious and wanting, needing, begging for information she went on a quest to get information, figure out how we could eat and survive without going into bankruptcy.

First and foremost, we started eating a lot and I mean a LOT of vegetables – cooked, raw, as a drink, whatever way she could think of, and trust me, she thought of things that sounded horrible, but ended up tasting great. Whoever thought beets, onions, carrots, spinach, apples, ginger and a banana would taste like a fruit drink? Not this guy!

Well, we are NOT the juicer type of people; we want to sink our teeth into some meat and potatoes from time to time, so we had to get back to some real food, although we still make and enjoy our homemade juice concoctions from time to time and cook some interesting (crazy) stuff.

Back *on* track…. We wanted some bread, like REALLY wanted some bread and finally found some GF bread and thought yes, yes, yes and even high fived each other…that is until we looked at the price. Now, regular breads are nice, fluffy, big loafs and they cost around $2, but the one we were holding fit in one hand, was frozen, only a few slices and cost $7.59, WHAT??????? WHY????????

So, now we were on another mission – a mission to save money and figure out how we could do that and eat decent food. We aren't the homemaker type that can make our own breads, and even then, GF flour costs much more as well. Everything costs more because it says "gluten free" or has the big GF emblem on it. Many think it's a fad and they want to cash in. For many, this isn't the case – it's a necessity and charging more for a medical condition is WRONG.

I have to admit, GF foods have gotten much better, there has been an explosion of GF products hitting the market and many aren't that bad, although beware, not everything that says GF actually is, as my wife yells, I mean tells me all the time, "Honey, read the label."

In studying and learning more everyday about gluten-free and doing research, I have learned there is a way to save money, not immediately, but when tax time comes. I can file and get money due to being GF. I thought to myself, "Why hasn't anyone shared this information? Why are people spending so much on GF and suffering when they can benefit in the end, not only with health, but finances as well?" This is never explained so everyone can understand it or it's just not explained properly. Here it is, in plain text, nothing hidden.

Number 1: Official Diagnosis – kind of like being in school and getting a doctor's note, stating you have a medical condition that states gluten-related disorder. This should also be in your records as part of the treatment plan. **Simply - a prescription from your doctor for a gluten free diet. (Too easy)**

Number 2: Save ALL grocery receipts that contain GF items. You will have to calculate the difference in food cost between gluten free and gluten-containing foods. You will be able to claim the difference between the two; for example, GF bread $7, bread with gluten $2, you can claim $5 as a difference. **What? WOW!**

Number 3: Fill out the medical deductions form, **Form 1040, Schedule A**, DO NOT fill out the short form as you won't be able to add the medical deductions.

Here are a couple of links you might find worth checking out:

http://www.beyondceliac.org/SiteData/docs/3ThingsYou/bfba5282a-0da53d2/3%20Things%20You%20Need%20to%20Know%20Before%20Filing%20Your%20Taxes.pdf

http://www.forbes.com/sites/kellyphillipserb/2016/09/02/back-to-school-tax-breaks-for-food-allergies-celiac-disease-other-special-diets/2/#47ab6304261c

https://celiac.org/celiac-disease/resources/government-benefits/tax-deductions-for-celiac-disease/

IRS Publication 502 provides that:

You can include in medical expenses amounts paid for admission and transportation to a medical conference if the medical conference concerns the chronic illness of yourself, your spouse, or dependent. The costs of the medical conference must be primarily for and necessary to the medical care of you, your spouse, or your dependent. The majority of the time spent at the conference must be spent attending sessions on medical information.

However, you may not deduct the costs for meals and lodging while attending the medical conference.

Read more at: https://celiac.org/celiac-disease/resources/government-benefits/tax-deductions-for-celiac-disease/#wFGZSJmzYkTjmue0.99

So, what are we offering in this book? We have made it easy for you to track your records and keep everything in order. We all know that shopping in itself can be a pain, and keeping receipts in order as well as tracking the price differences can really add to the headache.

We made it simple and easy. In this book there is a 52 page ledger for the 52 weeks of the year with a few extra pages to meet whatever shopping needs you may have. Whenever you go shopping, put the cost of your GF items down immediately on your tracker. Also put the average price of the product containing gluten, subtract the difference and there you go. Once you have completed the weeks' worth of shopping, add up the total amounts and see what you could be recouping once you file your taxes.

Remember, everyone has rights within the law and we need to hold someone accountable for the outrageous prices for GF foods. If it comes down to our government having to pay the difference, so be it – this is our lives, not a game and we deserve to eat healthy and not be in the poorhouse because of it.

There is an example page to show the differences and how to figure your total cost. Now go save yourself some money and be gluten-free without all the cost.

Enjoy gluten-free, saving money and have a healthy and happy life,

Ken and Katherine Henry (GF)

GF Tax Relief
Sample Page

Date	Store	Mileage	Product	GF	Gluten	Size Difference	Amount per Difference	Price Difference
22-Oct-16	Local	14	Pizza	10oz 7.99	20oz 3.89	10oz	.79 / .19 per oz	$4.10
23-Oct-16	Local	14	Frozen Burrito	3.49 ea	89 ea	same		$2.60
1-Nov-16	Local	14	Fish Sticks	14oz 8.99	19oz 4.79	5oz	.64 / .25 per oz	$5.00
5-Nov-16	Local	14	Chicken Nuggets	14oz 8.99	28oz 3.99	5oz	.64 / .14 per oz	$5.00
5-Nov-16	Local	14	Donuts (Frozen)	4ct 5.99	6ct 2.99	2ct	1.5 / .50 ea	$3.00
5-Nov-16	Local	14	Waffles	10oz 3.29	29oz 3.79	19oz	.33 / .13 per oz	$0.50
5-Nov-16	Local	14	Biscuits	4ct 7.39	10ct .50	6ct	1.98 / .05 ea	$6.89
5-Nov-16	Local	14	Pie Crust	2ct 4.99	2ct 2.19	same	2.50 / 1.09 ea	$2.80
5-Nov-16	Local	14	Bread (Shelf)	14oz 5.59	14oz .99	same	.40 / .07 per oz	$4.60
5-Nov-16	Local	14	English Muffin	6ct 5.99	18ct 2.99	12ct	1.00 / .37 ea	$3.00
5-Nov-16	Local	14	Cheesecake	14oz 6.99	17oz 4.44	3oz	.50 / .26 per oz	$2.55
5-Nov-16	Local	14	Tortilla	6ct 3.79	20ct 2.99	14ct	.63 / .14 ea	$0.80
5-Nov-16	Local	14	Baguettes	2ct 7.39	2ct 1.99	same	3.70 / .99 ea	$5.40
5-Nov-16	Local	14	Cereal	8oz 6.99	18oz 2.49	10oz	.87 / .14 per oz	$4.50
5-Nov-16	Local	14	Granola	10oz 6.99	11oz 2.95	1oz	.69 / .27 per oz	$4.04
5-Nov-16	Local	14	Peanut Butter	16oz 11.99	16oz 1.99	same	.75 / .12 per oz	$10.00
5-Nov-16	Local	14	Sugar Cookies Mix	12oz 3.99	17oz 2.00	5oz	.33 / .12 per oz	$1.99
5-Nov-16	Local	14	Muffin Mix	12oz 3.99	17oz 2.00	5oz	.33 / .12 per oz	$1.99
5-Nov-16	Local	14	Macaroni and cheese	6oz 2.99	7.25oz 1.30	1.25oz	.50 / .18 per oz	$1.69
5-Nov-16	Local	14	Wild Rice	8oz 6.79	16oz 1.19	8oz	.85 / .07 per oz	$5.60
5-Nov-16	Local	14	Cup of Noodles	1.1oz 1.99	2.25oz .35	1.15oz	1.81 / .15 per oz	$1.64
5-Nov-16	Local	14	Vanilla Wafers	6.3oz 4.19	11oz 2.59	4.7oz	.67 / .24 per oz	$1.60
4-Dec-16	Local	14	Honey Grahams	7.5oz 4.29	14.4oz 2.29	6.9oz	.57 / .15 per oz	$2.00
4-Dec-16	Local	14	Cookies	8oz 4.99	12oz 2.00	4oz	.62 / .17 per oz	$2.99
4-Dec-16	Local	14	Fig Bars	9oz 4.89	10oz 2.99	1oz	.54 / .29 per oz	$1.90
4-Dec-16	Local	14	Crackers	4oz 3.99	15oz 1.79	11oz	1.00 / .12 per oz	$2.20
4-Dec-16	Local	14	Flour	3lbs 16.99	5lbs 1.69	2lbs	5.66 / .34 per lb	$15.30
4-Dec-16	Local	14	Spaghetti	12oz 2.29	16oz .79	4oz	.19 / .04 per oz	$1.50
4-Dec-16	Local	14	Hamburger Buns	4ct 4.99	12ct 1.99	8ct	1.25 / .17 ea	$3.00
4-Dec-16	Local	14	Hotdog Buns	4ct 4.99	8ct 1.29	4ct	1.25 / .16 ea	$3.70
		TOTAL		TOTAL	TOTAL			TOTAL Diff.
		70		$184.20	$77.09			$107.11

Date	Store	Mileage	Product	GF Cost	Gluten Cost	Price Difference
		Total Miles		Total Cost	Total Cost	Price Difference

Date	Store	Mileage	Product	GF Cost	Gluten Cost	Price Difference
		Total Miles		Total Cost	Total Cost	Price Difference

Date	Store	Mileage	Product	GF Cost	Gluten Cost	Price Difference
		Total Miles		Total Cost	Total Cost	Price Difference

Date	Store	Mileage	Product	GF Cost	Gluten Cost	Price Difference
		Total Miles		Total Cost	Total Cost	Price Difference

Date	Store	Mileage	Product	GF Cost	Gluten Cost	Price Difference
		Total Miles		Total Cost	Total Cost	Price Difference

Date	Store	Mileage	Product	GF Cost	Gluten Cost	Price Difference
		Total Miles		Total Cost	Total Cost	Price Difference

Date	Store	Mileage	Product	GF Cost	Gluten Cost	Price Difference
		Total Miles		Total Cost	Total Cost	Price Difference

Date	Store	Mileage	Product	GF Cost	Gluten Cost	Price Difference
		Total Miles		Total Cost	Total Cost	Price Difference

Date	Store	Mileage	Product	GF Cost	Gluten Cost	Price Difference
		Total Miles		Total Cost	Total Cost	Price Difference

Date	Store	Mileage	Product	GF Cost	Gluten Cost	Price Difference
		Total Miles		Total Cost	Total Cost	Price Difference

Date	Store	Mileage	Product	GF Cost	Gluten Cost	Price Difference
		Total Miles		Total Cost	Total Cost	Price Difference

Date	Store	Mileage	Product	GF Cost	Gluten Cost	Price Difference
		Total Miles		Total Cost	Total Cost	Price Difference

Date	Store	Mileage	Product	GF Cost	Gluten Cost	Price Difference
		Total Miles		Total Cost	Total Cost	Price Difference

Date	Store	Mileage	Product	GF Cost	Gluten Cost	Price Difference
		Total Miles		Total Cost	Total Cost	Price Difference

Date	Store	Mileage	Product	GF Cost	Gluten Cost	Price Difference
		Total Miles		Total Cost	Total Cost	Price Difference

Date	Store	Mileage	Product	GF Cost	Gluten Cost	Price Difference
		Total Miles		Total Cost	Total Cost	Price Difference

Date	Store	Mileage	Product	GF Cost	Gluten Cost	Price Difference
		Total Miles		Total Cost	Total Cost	Price Difference

Date	Store	Mileage	Product	GF Cost	Gluten Cost	Price Difference
		Total Miles		Total Cost	Total Cost	Price Difference

Date	Store	Mileage	Product	GF Cost	Gluten Cost	Price Difference
		Total Miles		Total Cost	Total Cost	Price Difference

Date	Store	Mileage	Product	GF Cost	Gluten Cost	Price Difference
	Total Miles			**Total Cost**	**Total Cost**	**Price Difference**

Date	Store	Mileage	Product	GF Cost	Gluten Cost	Price Difference
		Total Miles		Total Cost	Total Cost	Price Difference

Date	Store	Mileage	Product	GF Cost	Gluten Cost	Price Difference
			Total Miles	Total Cost	Total Cost	Price Difference

Date	Store	Mileage	Product	GF Cost	Gluten Cost	Price Difference
		Total Miles		Total Cost	Total Cost	Price Difference

Date	Store	Mileage	Product	GF Cost	Gluten Cost	Price Difference
		Total Miles		Total Cost	Total Cost	Price Difference

Date	Store	Mileage	Product	GF Cost	Gluten Cost	Price Difference
		Total Miles		Total Cost	Total Cost	Price Difference

Date	Store	Mileage	Product	GF Cost	Gluten Cost	Price Difference
		Total Miles		Total Cost	Total Cost	Price Difference

Date	Store	Mileage	Product	GF Cost	Gluten Cost	Price Difference
		Total Miles		Total Cost	Total Cost	Price Difference

Date	Store	Mileage	Product	GF Cost	Gluten Cost	Price Difference
		Total Miles		Total Cost	Total Cost	Price Difference

Date	Store	Mileage	Product	GF Cost	Gluten Cost	Price Difference
		Total Miles		Total Cost	Total Cost	Price Difference

Date	Store	Mileage	Product	GF Cost	Gluten Cost	Price Difference
		Total Miles		Total Cost	Total Cost	Price Difference

Date	Store	Mileage	Product	GF Cost	Gluten Cost	Price Difference
		Total Miles		Total Cost	Total Cost	Price Difference

Date	Store	Mileage	Product	GF Cost	Gluten Cost	Price Difference
		Total Miles		Total Cost	Total Cost	Price Difference

Date	Store	Mileage	Product	GF Cost	Gluten Cost	Price Difference
		Total Miles		Total Cost	Total Cost	Price Difference

Date	Store	Mileage	Product	GF Cost	Gluten Cost	Price Difference
		Total Miles		Total Cost	Total Cost	Price Difference

Date	Store	Mileage	Product	GF Cost	Gluten Cost	Price Difference
		Total Miles		Total Cost	Total Cost	Price Difference

Date	Store	Mileage	Product	GF Cost	Gluten Cost	Price Difference
		Total Miles		Total Cost	Total Cost	Price Difference

Date	Store	Mileage	Product	GF Cost	Gluten Cost	Price Difference
		Total Miles		Total Cost	Total Cost	Price Difference

Date	Store	Mileage	Product	GF Cost	Gluten Cost	Price Difference
		Total Miles		Total Cost	Total Cost	Price Difference

Date	Store	Mileage	Product	GF Cost	Gluten Cost	Price Difference
		Total Miles		Total Cost	Total Cost	Price Difference

Date	Store	Mileage	Product	GF Cost	Gluten Cost	Price Difference
		Total Miles		Total Cost	Total Cost	Price Difference

Date	Store	Mileage	Product	GF Cost	Gluten Cost	Price Difference
		Total Miles		Total Cost	Total Cost	Price Difference

Date	Store	Mileage	Product	GF Cost	Gluten Cost	Price Difference
		Total Miles		Total Cost	Total Cost	Price Difference

Date	Store	Mileage	Product	GF Cost	Gluten Cost	Price Difference
		Total Miles		Total Cost	Total Cost	Price Difference

Date	Store	Mileage	Product	GF Cost	Gluten Cost	Price Difference
		Total Miles		Total Cost	Total Cost	Price Difference

Date													
Store													
Mileage											Total Miles		
Product													
GF Cost											Total Cost		
Gluten Cost											Total Cost		
Price Difference											Price Difference		

Date	Store	Mileage	Product	GF Cost	Gluten Cost	Price Difference
		Total Miles		Total Cost	Total Cost	Price Difference

Date	Store	Mileage	Product	GF Cost	Gluten Cost	Price Difference
		Total Miles		Total Cost	Total Cost	Price Difference

Date	Store	Mileage	Product	GF Cost	Gluten Cost	Price Difference
		Total Miles		Total Cost	Total Cost	Price Difference

Date	Store	Mileage	Product	GF Cost	Gluten Cost	Price Difference
		Total Miles		Total Cost	Total Cost	Price Difference

Date	Store	Mileage	Product	GF Cost	Gluten Cost	Price Difference
		Total Miles		Total Cost	Total Cost	Price Difference

Date	Store	Mileage	Product	GF Cost	Gluten Cost	Price Difference
		Total Miles		Total Cost	Total Cost	Price Difference

Date	Store	Mileage	Product	GF Cost	Gluten Cost	Price Difference
		Total Miles		Total Cost	Total Cost	Price Difference

Date	Store	Mileage	Product	GF Cost	Gluten Cost	Price Difference
		Total Miles		Total Cost	Total Cost	Price Difference

Date	Store	Mileage	Product	GF Cost	Gluten Cost	Price Difference
		Total Miles		Total Cost	Total Cost	Price Difference

Date	Store	Mileage	Product	GF Cost	Gluten Cost	Price Difference
		Total Miles		Total Cost	Total Cost	Price Difference

Date	Store	Mileage	Product	GF Cost	Gluten Cost	Price Difference
		Total Miles		Total Cost	Total Cost	Price Difference

Date	Store	Mileage	Product	GF Cost	Gluten Cost	Price Difference
		Total Miles		Total Cost	Total Cost	Price Difference

Date	Store	Mileage	Product	GF Cost	Gluten Cost	Price Difference
		Total Miles		Total Cost	Total Cost	Price Difference

Week	Mileage Totals	GF Cost Totals	Gluten Cost Totals	Cost Difference
1				
2				
3				
4				
5				
6				
7				
8				
9				
10				
11				
12				
13				
14				
15				
16				
17				
18				
19				
20				
Totals Weeks 1-20				

Week	Mileage Totals	GF Cost Totals	Gluten Cost Totals	Cost Difference
21				
22				
23				
24				
25				
26				
27				
28				
29				
30				
31				
32				
33				
34				
35				
36				
37				
38				
39				
40				
Totals Weeks 21-40				

Week	Mileage Totals	GF Cost Totals	Gluten Cost Totals	Cost Difference
41				
42				
43				
44				
45				
46				
47				
48				
49				
50				
51				
52				
Totals Weeks 21-52				
Weeks 1-20				
Weeks 21-40				
Weeks 41-52				
Annual Totals				

NATIONAL DEDICATED GLUTEN-FREE FOOD COMPANIES

UDI'S GLUTEN-FREE

http://udisglutenfree.com/products

PAMELA'S PRODUCTS

http://www.pamelasproducts.com/Products_frames.html

KINNIKINNICK

http://www.kinnikinnick.com/

SCHAR

http://www.schar.com/us/gluten-free-products/

GLUTINO

http://www.glutino.com/our-products/

WHOLE FOODS BAKEHOUSE

http://www.wholefoodsmarket.com/products/gluten-free-products.php

BOB'S RED MILL

http://www.bobsredmill.com/gluten-free/

AGAINST THE GRAIN GOURMET

http://www.againstthegraingourmet.com/

ENJOY LIFE FOODS

http://www.enjoylifefoods.com/our_foods/

CHEBE

http://www.chebe.com/

GLUTENFREEDA FOODS

http://www.glutenfreedafoods.com/

DEDICATED GLUTEN-FREE PRODUCT LINES

GENERAL MILLS GLUTEN-FREE LIST & WEBSITE

http://www.liveglutenfreely.com/products/

KING ARTHUR FLOUR GLUTEN-FREE PRODUCTS

http://www.kingarthurflour.com/glutenfree/

GLUTEN-FREE CAFE GLUTEN-FREE LIST

http://www.myglutenfreecafe.com/products

BIONATURAE GLUTEN-FREE PASTA

http://www.bionaturae.com/gluten.html

AMY'S GLUTEN-FREE PRODUCT LIST

http://www.amyskitchen.com/special_diets/celiac.php

ANNIE'S GLUTEN-FREE

http://www.annies.com/glutenfree

HODGSON MILL GLUTEN-FREE LIST

http://www.hodgsonmill.com/roi/673/Naturally-Gluten-Free-Products/

NATURE'S PATH GLUTEN-FREE ITEMS

http://www.naturespath.com/eat-well/gluten-free-celiac-diet

SAN-J GLUTEN-FREE ITEMS

http://www.san-j.com/faq.asp?#15

IAN'S NATURALS GLUTEN-FREE ITEMS

http://www.iansnaturalfoods.com/allergen_free.html

RUDI'S GLUTEN-FREE

http://www.rudisbakery.com/gluten-free/

LISTING OF FOOD THAT HAPPENS TO BE GLUTEN-FREE:

ANNIES NATURALS GLUTEN-FREE LIST
http://anniesnaturals.com/gluten_free

BOAR'S HEAD GLUTEN-FREE LIST
http://www.boarshead.com/gluten_free.php

CAMPBELL'S GLUTEN-FREE LIST
http://www.campbellsoupcompany.com/pdf/FAQ_GlutenFreeProductList.pdf

EDEN ORGANIC GLUTEN-FREE LIST
http://www.edenfoods.com/articles/view.php?articles_id=85

HAIN-CELESTIAL GLUTEN-FREE SITE
http://www.hain-celestial.com/gluten-free/index.php

HEINZ GLUTEN-FREE LIST
http://www.heinz.com/glutenfree/products.html

HORMEL GLUTEN-FREE LIST
http://www.hormelfoods.com/brands/glutenfree/default.aspx

LUNDBERG FARMS GLUTEN-FREE LIST
http://www.lundberg.com/Products/Special_diets/Glutenfree.aspx

MARZETTI GLUTEN-FREE LIST
http://www.marzetti.com/pdfs/faq/GlutenFreeList92710.pdf

NESTLE GLUTEN-FREE LIST
http://nestle-consumerservices.casupport.com/eglutenfree.pdf

ORGANIC VALLEY GLUTEN-FREE LIST
http://www.organicvalley.coop/products/gluten-free-products/

SNYDER'S OF HANOVER GLUTEN-FREE LIST
http://snydersofhanover.stores.yahoo.net/glfrprli.html

FRITO LAY GLUTEN-FREE LIST
http://www.fritolay.com/your-health/us-products-not-containing-gluten-in-gredients.html

ARROWHEAD MILLS GLUTEN-FREE PRODUCTS http://www.arrow-headmills.com/category/gluten-free

OTHER GLUTEN-FREE LINKS OF INTEREST

http://www.pilgrimspride.com/products/glutenfree.aspx

http://www.larabar.com/food/gluten-free-info

http://www.minuterice.com/en-us/products/full_allergy.aspx

http://www.immaculatebaking.com/products.php?id=17

http://www.jonesdairyfarm.com/Gluten-Free-C36.aspx

http://www.thaikitchen.com/Allergy-Information.aspx

Q & A

Q: Why are gluten free (GF) foods so much more expensive?

A: One of the reasons gluten-free foods are more expensive lies in the fact that cross-contamination is always a possibility. Therefore, bakeries producing products labeled gluten-free must pay to have the facilities thoroughly cleaned on a regular basis. They must also make their products in a facility that is dedicated to the highest standards. Moreover, every batch should be tested for allergy reasons. Additional staffing, special equipment and these additional steps are just a few of the reasons gluten-free foods come with a higher price tag than other foods.

High Cost/Low Competition: Overall, reports show that creating gluten-free foods can be 242% more costly than manufacturing products with less strict guidelines. Given this information, in conjunction with the fact that many manufacturers are not eager to sell gluten-free foods for this very reason, and it becomes abundantly clear not only why gluten free foods are more costly, but also that they're worth every penny.

Gluten Free Certifications: Another reason why gluten-free foods tend to cost more is because of the number of certifications required to bear the gluten-free label. These may include one or more of the following:

Gluten-Free Certification Organization (GFCO): GFCO is a certification program for the Gluten Intolerance Group® (GIG) that has been in place for several years for the aid of people with gluten intolerance symptoms. For a product to be labeled gluten-free, the level of gluten must be less than 10ppm, determined by third-party testing.

National Foundation for Celiac Awareness Gluten-Free Certification Program (NFCA): Products are certified gluten-free, according to NFCA, at 10ppm; however, all the raw ingredients in the product need to be tested and can be used only when their levels are less than 20ppm. A third-party check is required to ensure the regulations are followed.

The International Certification Services (ICS): Certified gluten-free standards help consumers make informed choices about foods to avoid because of gluten. Compliance with this standard involves a combination of analysis of the products and ingredients used in manufacturing and management practices that prevent introduction of gluten to the foods at any point in the manufacturing process. All products certified under this standard can be from one ingredient or a formula involving several ingredients.

Celiac Sprue Association Seal of Recognition (CSA): To receive certification from CSA, the gluten level in the product must be below 5ppm. In addition, products may not contain oats, as some people who react even if the oats have been certified gluten-free. This certification also does not allow the use of any ingredient that has gluten, even if the final product satisfies the 5ppm specification. Auditing and testing by a third party are required.

Gluten-Free Standards Organization (GFSA): If a manufactured product undergoes higher testing and the gluten level is less than 20ppm, then the manufacturer may display a special logo on the product. Full certification from GFSA, however, requires products to have gluten levels less than 3ppm.

Each one of these agencies has their own set of strict guidelines that can be time consuming and costly.

Q: Why are GF foods so hard to locate?

A: It's getting better as more stores are starting to carry gluten-free items, and they also have request forms to fill out asking for products to be carried locally. Gluten-free product companies also have request forms that will get them into stores if you ask the company themselves, they will send the request out. Online ordering is becoming huge and everything can be bought online these days, but staple foods must be bought off the shelf to save cost. Since some of these products are frozen, the shipping can be more costly and makes it not worth the cost – until now that is, now that you have the knowledge of retrieving monies back via taxes.

Q: Is there any way to save money and eat GF?

A: Yes, keep the ledger we provided along with envelopes for each month with your receipts in them. At the end of the year when you file your taxes, remember to file long form and use your numbers. You do NOT need to include receipts with your form, but DO keep in case you get audited, as this is your proof of purchase and cost differences.

Q & A SHORT AND SWEET

Q: <u>What is gluten?</u>
A: Storage proteins found in grains

Q: What types of gluten-related disorders are there?
A: Celiac disease or gluten sensitivity

Q: What is celiac disease?
A: An autoimmune disorder

Q: Why is celiac disease so serious?
A: It damages the small intestine

Q: How is celiac disease diagnosed?
A: Blood tests, skin biopsies and endoscopy

Q: What is gluten sensitivity?
A: Body responding from ingesting gluten

Q: What are some symptoms of gluten sensitivity?
A: Gastrointestinal problems, rash, or fatigue

Q: How is it diagnosed?
A: It's a "rule out" condition.

Q: Will I miss out on important nutrients?
A: No, you should absorb more.

Q: Why would I absorb more nutrients without gluten?
A: Gluten can inhibit nutrient absorption.

Q: It is low calorie?
A: Not always

Q: Can I still enjoy foods I love?
A: With some creativity and effort there is always a way

Q: Will it help me lose weight?
A: Yes, definitely a possibility

Q: Why do some people gain weight on GF?
A: Fillers in processed GF foods

Q: Can cutting out gluten be harmful?
A: Not with a balanced diet

Q: So what can I eat?
A: Fruits, vegetables, meat, dairy, nuts, GF breads, GF pasta

Q: Is it expensive?
A: It can be very expensive, definitely shop prices

Q: Can I still eat out?
A: Most restaurants will make accommodations. (Ensure they understand this isn't a "fad" diet and you have medical conditions).

Q: Will I be starving?
A: No, cravings are reduced.

Q: Will I have less energy?

A: Your energy levels will actually go up.

Q: Will it give me a flatter stomach?

A: It can reduce bloating.

Q: What's a non-gut related benefit of cutting out on gluten?

A: Less joint pain

Q: Will I lose fat?

A: Science says yes.

Q: Is Soy Sauce GF?

A: No. It's made with fermented wheat. <u>**BUT**</u>, Tamari makes a GF Soy Sauce that actually tastes better than regular, and there are quite a few more out there, read the labels.

Q: But salad's GF right?

A: The dressing may not be, again read labels

Q: Are gluten-free pastas better for me?

A: Pasta is pasta, there are so many types of GF pasta's out there, everything from bean to green.

Q: Is gluten related to emotional health?

A: Gluten sensitivity can cause depression!!

Q: Where do I shop?

A: Any grocery store that carries GF products or online

Q: What are GF "safe" brands?
A: GF whole foods, there are many "safe" brands out there, many listed above

Q: Is it hard?
A: It's certainly an adjustment, but once adjusted it comes pretty easy

Q: What are non-gluten grains?
A: Buckwheat, quinoa, sorghum, rice, millet

Q: Aren't oats gluten-free?
A: Cross-contamination is common, definitely read the labels on any oat products

Q: Is GF a fad?
A: Name a diet that isn't a fad at one time or another. Yes, it's a fad for some, for others, **NO**; it's a lifestyle of choice or medical condition

Q: What's the most important thing to remember?
A: READ THE LABEL / RESEARCH

FINAL WORDS

This book has been put together with lots of research, love, and hopes to help others since we understand the struggle.

Gluten-free to some is a fad diet that will pass, but for others it's a lifestyle or medical condition that requires us to cut out gluten.

Remember, you are not alone in your struggle. There are websites dedicated to gluten-free and there are people with the same issues that understand what you are going through and are willing to lend a hand.

Talk to people when shopping. When you see someone buy something gluten-free, strike up a conversation. This is how we found out about a lot of products we'd never heard of before – word of mouth is a powerful tool.

Gluten-free trade shows are an excellent way to learn about and try new products before you buy them. Plus they hand out lots of coupons, information and samples, and who doesn't love a good free sample before buying a product.

SO… Keep a ledger, save receipts in monthly envelopes, file long form, save money and enjoy your gluten-free life!!!!

Ken & Katherine Henry (GF)

NOTES

NOTES

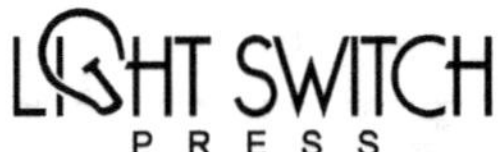

9 781944 255398